BOOST YOUR IMMUNITY

A PROFESSIONAL GUIDE

A.D RAMS

Contents

CHAPTER ONE 3

INTRODUCTION 3

   The Value of Immune Function 7

   Knowledge of the Immune System 12

   Lifestyle Variables Affecting Immune Function........17

CHAPTER TWO 22

   Nutritional Techniques to Boost Immunity............22

   Physical Activity and Immunity 28

   Getting Enough Sleep to Boost Immunity...............33

   Techniques for Stress Management 39

   Cleanliness and Immune Defense 44

CHAPTER THREE 46

   Immune support and supplements.........................50

   Immune Functioning Throughout Life 55

   CONCLUSION...61

THE END 65

CHAPTER ONE

INTRODUCTION

Improving immunity is essential to preserving general health and wellbeing. Our immune system defends our bodies from a range of diseases and infections by acting as a barrier against dangerous organisms such as bacteria, viruses, and toxins. Immune function is influenced by a variety of lifestyle factors in addition to genetics, including nutrition, exercise, sleep patterns, stress reduction, and personal hygiene.

Developing immune-supporting and immune-stiffening behaviors is part of knowing how to increase immunity. Here's a quick rundown of different methods to increase immunity:

Healthy Diet: Immune system performance depends on consuming a balanced diet high in vitamins, minerals, antioxidants, and other nutrients. To ensure that your body gets all the nutrients it needs, make sure your meals include an abundance of fruits, vegetables, whole grains, lean proteins, and healthy fats.

Frequent Exercise: By encouraging healthy circulation, lowering inflammation, and bolstering general health, regular physical activity can improve immune function. On most days of the week, try to get in at least 30 minutes of moderate activity.

Sufficient Sleep: Immune system performance and general health depend on getting enough good sleep. Try to get between 7 and 9 hours of sleep every night to give your body time to relax, heal, and replenish.

Stress management: Over time, persistent stress might impair immunity. To encourage resilience and relaxation, try stress-reduction methods like yoga, deep breathing exercises, mindfulness meditation, or spending time in nature.

Hygiene Practices: Good hygiene helps lower the risk of illness and stop the transmission of infectious diseases. This includes regularly washing your hands with soap and water.

Reducing Alcohol and Tobacco Use: Smoking and excessive alcohol use can weaken the immune system and make people more vulnerable to illnesses. Reducing or staying away from these chemicals can assist in maintaining a strong immune system.

Supplements: Certain supplements, including probiotics, zinc, vitamin C, and vitamin D, may assist support immune function in certain situations, particularly in those with immune system shortages or compromises. However, before beginning any new supplement regimen, it is imperative to speak with a healthcare provider.

You may boost your immunity and lower your chance of disease by implementing these techniques into your everyday practice. Recall that the secret to long-term immunological health and general wellbeing is to maintain a healthy lifestyle.

The Value of Immune Function

It is impossible to overestimate the significance of immunological health because the immune system is essential for both defending the body against infections and preserving general health. The following are some main arguments in favor of immune system health:

Disease Prevention: The body's first line of defense against diseases brought on by bacteria, fungi, viruses, and other pathogens is a strong immune system. By locating and eliminating these intruders before they have a chance to spread sickness, it lowers the chance of contracting infectious diseases including the common cold, the flu, pneumonia, and more serious infections.

Faster Recovery: The body recovers from diseases and infections more quickly when its immune system is operating at peak performance, which allows it to identify and get rid of germs more quickly. Reducing the intensity of symptoms can also be aided by a robust immunological response.

Protection Against Chronic Diseases: The immune system is essential for the prevention and management of chronic diseases including cancer, autoimmune disorders, and metabolic disorders like diabetes, in addition to warding off acute infections. An intact immune system can aid in controlling inflammation and preventing the onset of certain illnesses.

General Health and Well-Being: General health and well-being are intimately related to immune function. A healthy immune system helps people feel resilient, alive, and full of energy, which makes it easier for them to handle stress and lead fulfilling lives.

Enhanced Longevity: Studies indicate that by lowering the danger of infectious illnesses and chronic ailments that can shorten life expectancy, immune system health may enhance longevity.

Enhanced immunological Response to Vaccinations: Vaccines can prevent a variety of infectious diseases, and an efficient immunological response to them depends on a healthy immune system. Vaccines elicit the production of memory cells and antibodies by the immune system, which offer sustained defense against particular diseases.

Improved Surgical Results: Immune system strength plays a major role in wound healing and infection prevention both before and after surgery. Individuals with weakened immune systems are more likely to experience difficulties following surgery and might need further medical care.

Protection During Aging: Due to natural immune system alterations brought on by aging, older folks are more vulnerable to infections and other health issues. It is possible to promote healthy aging and lower the risk of age-related diseases by maintaining immunological health through lifestyle choices and preventative actions.

Maintaining overall health, energy, and resilience throughout life requires prioritizing immune health through good lifestyle choices, appropriate nutrition, regular exercise, enough sleep, stress management, and preventive healthcare measures. Putting money into immunological health is an investment in one's quality of life and long-term wellbeing.

The immune system is an intricate network of tissues, cells, and organs that cooperate to protect the body from pathogens such bacteria, fungi, viruses, and parasites. Its major job is to differentiate between non-self (things that are not part of the body) and self (the body's own cells and tissues), and to get rid of the non-self invaders while preserving tolerance for the self-components. An outline of the immune system's main elements and operations is provided below:

Nonspecific immunity, also referred to as innate immunity, is the immune system's ability to defend the body against infections without the need for previous exposure. It is the initial line of defense and consists of cellular elements like neutrophils, macrophages, natural killer (NK) cells, complement proteins, and mucous membranes as well as physical barriers like the skin. Although innate immunity is not pathogen-specific, it reacts quickly to infection and inflammation.

Adaptive Immunity: Also referred to as acquired immunity, this immune system matures more slowly but offers a sustained and focused defense against particular infections. It involves specialized cells called T cells and B cells, which go through maturation and activation processes in order to identify and get rid of particular antigens, which are chemicals found on the surface of pathogens. B cells' generation of antibodies and the activation of cytotoxic T cells, which destroy infected cells directly, are two aspects of the adaptive immune response.

Lymphoid Organs: The bone marrow, thymus, spleen, lymph nodes, tonsils, and mucosa-associated lymphoid tissue (MALT) are among the specialized organs and tissues where the immune system predominantly functions. These organs perform the functions of lymphatic and blood filtering, which eliminates infections and foreign particles, as well as immune cell formation, maturation, and interaction.

Immune cells create signaling chemicals called chemokines and cytokines, which promote cell division, development, migration, and communication in order to control the immune response. In order to control inflammation and immunological responses, as well as to coordinate the activity of immune cells, cytokines and chemokines are crucial.

Memory and Immunological Memory: The adaptive immune system's capacity to develop immunological memory is one of its most amazing traits. Memory T cells and B cells are produced in response to exposure to a particular pathogen or antigen, offering sustained protection against reinfection. When the immune system comes into contact with the same virus again, it will be able to mount a stronger and quicker defense because to this memory response.

Tolerance Mechanisms: To prevent autoimmune reactions, the immune system needs to be able to tolerate the body's own cells and tissues in addition to protecting against external threats. Immune homeostasis is preserved and inappropriate immune responses against self-antigens are suppressed with the aid of regulatory T cells (Tregs) and other systems.

All things considered, the immune system is an extremely complex and dynamic defensive mechanism that keeps an eye out for any indications of infection or anomaly, mounts the proper defenses to get rid of dangers, and strikes a careful balance between self-tolerance and protective immunity. In order to improve immune health, prevent disease, and treat immunological-related problems, it is imperative to comprehend the structure and function of the immune system.

Lifestyle Variables Affecting Immune Function

Numerous lifestyle choices have a major impact on immunological function, either favorably or unfavorably. Through the adoption of beneficial habits and the avoidance of harmful ones, people can enhance their immune system and lessen their vulnerability to illnesses and infections. The following are important lifestyle choices that affect immune function:

Diet: Maintaining a strong immune system requires adequate nutrition. A balanced diet that includes whole grains, fruits, vegetables, lean meats, healthy fats, and other nutrients is the best way to receive the vitamins, minerals, antioxidants, and other nutrients your immune system needs. Important minerals include iron, zinc, selenium, vitamin C, vitamin D, and vitamin E.

Hydration: Keeping the immune system operating at its best requires proper hydration. Water facilitates the uptake of nutrients by cells, eliminates toxins from the body, and supports the healthy operation of immune cells. Try to stay hydrated during the day by drinking lots of water and avoiding sugar-filled drinks and too much coffee, which can diuretic.

Exercise: Research has shown that immune function can be improved by regular physical activity because it improves circulation, lowers inflammation, and supports general health. Almost every day of the week, moderate-intensity exercise can boost immunity and lower the chance of infection. But too much or too strenuous exercise might temporarily impair immune function, so moderation is key.

Sleep: Since it enables the body to rest, heal, and rebuild, getting enough quality sleep is essential for immune system function. The immune system fights against infections by releasing defensive chemicals including cytokines as you sleep. To boost immune function, aim for 7-9 hours of sleep each night and create a regular sleep regimen.

Handling Stress: Prolonged stress can impair immunity and make a person more vulnerable to illnesses and infections. To encourage resilience and relaxation, try stress-reduction methods like yoga, deep breathing exercises, mindfulness meditation, or spending time in nature. Immune health can be supported by making self-care a priority and developing good coping strategies for stressful situations.

cleanliness Practices: Keeping the immune system strong and halting the spread of infectious diseases depend heavily on good cleanliness. Frequently wash your hands with soap and water, particularly either before or right after using the restroom, coughing, or sneezing. When coughing or sneezing, cover your mouth and nose as a sign of excellent respiratory hygiene and stay away from people who are unwell.

Reducing Alcohol and Tobacco Use: Smoking and excessive alcohol use can weaken the immune system and make people more vulnerable to illnesses. Reducing or eliminating these compounds can lower the risk of respiratory infections, cardiovascular disorders, and other health issues while also supporting a strong immune system.

Social Network: Having a strong support system and strong social ties can have a good impact on immunological function.

CHAPTER TWO

Research has indicated that those with strong social support networks typically have higher immune systems and general health. Schedule quality time for socializing with loved ones, friends, and neighbors.

You may encourage general health and well-being, lower your risk of illness, and boost and improve your immune system by implementing these lifestyle variables into your daily routine.

Nutritional Techniques to Boost Immunity

Nutritional techniques are essential for maintaining general health and immune system performance. People can boost their immunity and lessen their vulnerability to illnesses by consuming meals high in vital nutrients and developing healthy eating habits. The following are some essential dietary tactics to boost immunity:

Eat a Balanced Diet: To maintain immune function, one must consume a well-rounded diet that contains a variety of nutrient-dense foods. To provide your body the vitamins, minerals, antioxidants, and other nutrients it needs, try to incorporate a balance of fruits, vegetables, whole grains, lean meats, and healthy fats in your meals.

Emphasis on Foods High in Antioxidants: Antioxidants aid in defending cells against oxidative stress and free radical damage, which can compromise immunological function. Consume a diet rich in foods high in antioxidants, such as almonds, tomatoes, bell peppers, cruciferous vegetables (like broccoli and kale), leafy greens, berries, citrus fruits, and kiwi.

Boost Your Vitamin C Intake: Vitamin C is well-known for strengthening the immune system and assisting in the development and operation of white blood cells, which are critical for warding off infections. Include foods high in vitamin C in your diet, such as broccoli, spinach, bell peppers, strawberries, kiwis, and citrus fruits (such as oranges and grapefruits).

Achieve Adequate Vitamin D: Vitamin D is essential for controlling immunological response and lowering the risk of respiratory infections. As your skin produces vitamin D in reaction to sunshine exposure, spend time outside. You may also increase your intake of vitamin D-rich foods by eating foods like eggs, dairy products, fortified cereals, and fatty fish (like salmon and mackerel).

Incorporate Foods High in Zinc: Zinc plays a role in several elements of immune function, including as the growth and operation of immune cells and the generation of antibodies. Consume foods high in zinc, such as whole grains, dairy products, beans, nuts, seeds, seafood (such as oysters, crab, and shrimp), and lean meats and poultry.

Eat Omega-3 Fatty Acids: These fats have anti-inflammatory qualities and may aid in immune system support. Consume foods high in omega-3 fatty acids, such as walnuts, hemp seeds, flaxseeds, chia seeds, and fatty fish (salmon, mackerel, and sardines).

Fermented foods with probiotics: Probiotics are good bacteria that support gut health and may strengthen the immune system. Eat foods high in probiotics, such as tempeh, yogurt, kefir, sauerkraut, kimchi, miso, and miso, to help maintain a balanced gut microbiome.

Keep Yourself Hydrated: Maintaining good health and immunological function requires adequate hydration. Water is the best beverage to consume throughout the day. Avoid high caffeine and sugary drinks since they may have a diuretic effect.

Restrict Your Intake of Processed Foods and Added Sugars: Consuming these foods and added sugars in excess can compromise your immune system and exacerbate inflammation in your body. Restrict your use of sugary snacks, sodas, processed meats, and refined carbohydrates. Whenever feasible, choose whole, less processed foods.

You can boost your immune system, lower your risk of infection, and improve your general health and well-being by implementing these dietary practices into your daily routine. It's important to keep in mind, though, that no single diet or ingredient can miraculously strengthen your immune system. Rather, concentrate on eating a well-balanced diet that is full of different nutrients to help your immune system work at its best.

Physical Activity and Immunity

The immune system and general wellbeing are greatly aided by exercise. Frequent exercise has been demonstrated to boost immunity in a number of ways, lowering the risk of infections and long-term illnesses. This is how immunological health is impacted by exercise:

Enhanced Immune Surveillance: Exercise increases immune cell circulation throughout the body, which improves the immune system's capacity to identify and get rid of diseases. By strengthening the body's defenses against infections, this may help lower the chance of infection.

Diminished Chronic Inflammation: Autoimmune diseases, cardiovascular diseases, and metabolic disorders are among the problems that are linked to chronic inflammation. Frequent exercise promotes a more balanced immune response and modulates the production of inflammatory markers, both of which contribute to the reduction of chronic inflammation.

Better Gut Health: Research indicates that exercise helps maintain a balanced gut flora, which is essential for immunological function. A well-balanced and varied gut microbiota has been linked to improved immunity and decreased vulnerability to infections and autoimmune disorders.

Stress Reduction: Engaging in physical activity can help lower levels of stress hormones like cortisol and adrenaline. Exercise as a stress management strategy can indirectly improve immunological health because long-term stress weakens the immune system and increases susceptibility to illnesses.

Enhanced Vaccine Response: Studies have demonstrated that regular exercise increases the body's generation of memory cells and antibodies, which improves the body's reaction to vaccinations. This can lower the risk of infections by triggering a stronger and longer-lasting immune response against particular bacteria.

Optimized Weight Management: Reducing the risk of obesity-related disorders like type 2 diabetes, cardiovascular diseases, and some malignancies can be achieved by maintaining a healthy weight through regular exercise. Since obesity is linked to weakened immune system and chronic inflammation, reaching and maintaining a healthy weight can help promote immune system health in general.

Better Lung Function and Strengthened Respiratory Muscles: Aerobic exercises, including brisk walking, jogging, or cycling, can enhance lung function and build respiratory muscles. This could lower the chance of respiratory infections and improve the body's resistance to respiratory ailments including pneumonia, the flu, and colds.

Improved Sleep Quality: Frequent exercise is linked to longer and better-quality sleep, which is crucial for immune system performance and general health. Sufficient sleep promotes optimum immune function and resilience against infections by allowing the body to relax, repair, and rejuvenate.

While moderate exercise helps strengthen the immune system, excessive or severe exercise can temporarily depress immune function. This is especially true if the activity is not balanced with enough rest and recuperation. As a result, it's critical to pay attention to your body, refrain from overtraining, and mix up your routine with a range of physical activities, such as flexibility exercises, strength training, cardiovascular activity, and relaxation methods. You can enhance immune function and advance general wellbeing by sticking to a regular, well-balanced workout schedule.

Getting Enough Sleep to Boost Immunity

Getting enough sleep is essential for maintaining immune system performance and general health. The body goes through a number of physiological changes when you sleep that are critical to preserving healthy immune system performance and infection resistance. Here's how getting enough sleep boosts immunity:

Sleep is necessary for the generation and operation of immune cells, such as natural killer (NK) cells, T cells, and white blood cells, all of which are vital for protecting the body from infections. Getting enough sleep makes it possible for the immune system to be primed and prepared to fight against threats.

Sleep aids in the regulation of the body's inflammatory response, which is necessary for warding off infections and promoting wound healing. Prolonged sleep deprivation can raise inflammation levels in the body, which can weaken the immune system and make people more prone to infections and long-term illnesses.

The production of cytokines, which are signaling molecules that control inflammation and immunological responses, occurs while you sleep. While sleep deprivation can upset this balance and result in dysregulated immune responses, enough sleep promotes the balanced synthesis of cytokines.

Enhanced Immune Reaction: Research has demonstrated that getting enough sleep helps the body react better to vaccinations by increasing the generation of memory cells and antibodies. This can lower the risk of infections by triggering a stronger and longer-lasting immune response against particular bacteria.

Sleep has an impact on the balance of the gut microbiota, which is essential for immunological function. Sleep disturbances or prolonged sleep deprivation can have a deleterious effect on the gut flora, which may jeopardize immunological health.

Stress Reduction: Getting enough sleep aids in the regulation of stress hormones like cortisol and adrenaline, which, when persistently raised, can have immunosuppressive effects. Well-being is enhanced by getting enough sleep, which lowers stress and encourages relaxation.

Wound Healing and Repair: Sleep is necessary for the body's renewal of cells, tissue repair, and wound healing. Growth hormones are released by the body when you sleep, which aid in tissue regeneration and repair and strengthen your immune system as a whole.

Take into account the following advice to enhance immunological function and encourage restful sleep:

Even on weekends, stick to a regular sleep routine by going to bed and waking up at the same times each day.

Establish a soothing nighttime ritual, such as reading a book or taking a warm bath, to let your body know when it's time to unwind.

Invest on a supportive mattress and pillows, and create a cool, quiet, and dark sleeping environment.

Limit your time spent in front of displays (such as TVs, PCs, and smartphones) before bed because the blue light they emit can interfere with your sleep cycle.

Alcohol, nicotine, and caffeine should be avoided right before bed because they can disrupt your sleep.

Exercise on a regular basis, but steer clear of strenuous activities right before bed since they can keep you awake and interfere with your ability to fall asleep.

To encourage relaxation and enhance the quality of your sleep, learn stress management strategies including journaling, deep breathing exercises, and mindfulness meditation.

You may boost your immune system, improve your general health, and lower your risk of infections and chronic diseases by making quality sleep a priority and developing appropriate sleeping habits.

Techniques for Stress Management

Since chronic stress can have a detrimental effect on many aspects of health, including immunological function, effective stress management practices are crucial for supporting both mental and physical well-being. Stress management techniques can help people deal with stressors more effectively and lessen the negative effects stress has on their bodies. Here are a few tried-and-true methods for reducing stress:

By concentrating on the current moment without passing judgment, mindfulness meditation helps people become more conscious of their thoughts, feelings, and sensations. Regular mindfulness meditation has been demonstrated to enhance general wellbeing and lower stress, anxiety, and depression.

Deep Breathing Exercises: Deep breathing techniques, like belly breathing and diaphragmatic breathing, can help lower stress levels and trigger the body's relaxation response. People can induce relaxation and de-stress by breathing deeply and slowly while concentrating on their breathing.

Progressive muscular Relaxation (PMR): PMR is a method of relaxation in which the body's muscular groups are systematically moved from one tense state to another. This technique eases tense muscles and encourages both mental and physical relaxation.

Yoga: Yoga promotes strength, flexibility, and relaxation by combining physical postures with mindfulness exercises and breath control. Frequent yoga practice has been demonstrated to lower stress, elevate mood, and promote general wellbeing.

Exercise: Getting your body moving might help you feel better by generating endorphins, which are your body's natural feel-good hormones. Regular exercise can help lower stress levels and encourage relaxation, whether it be walking, jogging, cycling, or dancing.

Journaling: Putting ideas, feelings, and experiences down on paper in a journal can help you process your feelings and see stressful circumstances from a different angle. Writing in a journal can aid in mental clarity, pattern recognition, and the development of coping mechanisms for stress management.

Spending Time in Nature: Research has demonstrated that spending time in the great outdoors may have a calming and relaxing effect on the body and mind, lowering stress levels and encouraging relaxation. Spending time in nature, whether it be through trekking, park walks, or just relaxing in a garden, can reduce stress and enhance wellbeing.

Social Support: Engaging in conversation with friends, family, or a network of supporters can offer emotional support and improve a person's ability to manage stress. A sense of connection and belonging can be fostered and feelings of isolation can be lessened by sharing experiences, emotions, and worries with others.

Establishing limits: Reducing emotions of overwhelm and stress can be achieved by learning to say no and establishing limits with regard to work, obligations, and relationships. Maintaining balance and wellbeing requires setting aside time for leisure and relaxation activities as well as prioritizing self-care.

Seeking expert Assistance: Consulting a therapist or counselor, or other mental health expert, might be helpful if stress becomes too much to handle. Therapy can help people handle stress more effectively and enhance their general mental health by giving them coping mechanisms, resources, and techniques.

It's critical to try out several stress-reduction strategies to see which ones are most effective for you. Combining these techniques into your daily routine can improve your ability to manage stress, lessen its negative effects on your health, and enhance your general wellbeing.

Cleanliness and Immune Defense

Sustaining immune function and preventing infections require maintaining proper hygiene habits. By limiting the transmission of dangerous organisms including bacteria, viruses, and fungi, proper hygiene lowers the risk of sickness and enhances general health. The following important hygiene habits can support immune system protection:

Hand washing: One of the best strategies to stop the transmission of infectious diseases is to wash your hands frequently. Especially before eating, after using the restroom, after coughing or sneezing, and after touching surfaces in public areas, wash your hands often for at least 20 seconds with soap and water. Use hand sanitizer with at least 60% alcohol if soap and water aren't accessible.

CHAPTER THREE

Maintain proper respiratory hygiene to stop the spread of respiratory illnesses such as COVID-19, the flu, and colds. When you cough or sneeze, cover your mouth and nose with a tissue or your elbow. Be sure to properly dispose of used tissues. Refrain from touching your face because this can spread viruses from infected surfaces to mucous membranes. This includes touching your mouth, nose, and eyes.

Surface Cleaning: To lower the chance of contamination, keep regularly touched surfaces clean and sterilised. Doorknobs, light switches, counters, and electronic equipment should all be routinely cleaned using an EPA-approved disinfectant. Particular attention should be paid to surfaces in areas with heavy usage and shared areas.

Food Safety: To avoid contracting foodborne illnesses, practice good food hygiene. Before consuming or cooking, wash fruits and vegetables well. To ensure that hazardous bacteria are killed, cook meats, poultry, shellfish, and eggs to the proper internal temperature. Keep raw and cooked foods apart to prevent cross-contamination when storing perishable goods.

Personal Hygiene: To stop the spread of illnesses, practice proper personal hygiene. To maintain a clean physique, take regular baths or showers and be sure to properly wash your hands after using the restroom. To avoid gum disease and tooth infections, practice good oral hygiene by brushing your teeth at least twice a day and flossing every day.

Preventing Close Contact with Sick People: If someone in your family or neighborhood has a communicable disease, take steps to keep them at a distance from you in order to lower the chance of transmission. Urge sick people to refrain from going to work or school until they are well enough to return, and advise them not to share personal belongings like towels, sheets, or utensils.

Hygiene While Traveling: Take additional care to keep yourself clean and stop the spread of illnesses when you're on the road. Use hand sanitizer, wash your hands often, and refrain from touching your face. Maintain social distance, wear a mask in confined or crowded areas, and heed travel warnings and local health recommendations.

You may lessen the load on your immune system, safeguard people from diseases, and enhance immune health and wellbeing by adopting certain hygiene habits into your everyday routine. Furthermore, keeping up with the most recent recommendations and guidelines for public health can assist you in making well-informed decisions to safeguard your community and yourself against infectious diseases.

Supplements can help maintain immune function, particularly when dietary choices or certain medical conditions affect nutrient levels. It's important to remember, though, that supplements should support a healthy lifestyle and balanced diet rather than take their place. The following supplements are frequently linked to immune support:

Vitamin C: Rich in antioxidants, vitamin C boosts the immune system by promoting the development and activity of white blood cells, which aid in the body's defense against infections. For those who are deficient in the vitamin or are experiencing high levels of stress, vitamin C supplements may be helpful, but it's usually better to obtain enough of it through diet, such as citrus fruits, strawberries, kiwis, bell peppers, and broccoli.

Vitamin D: Vitamin D is essential for controlling immunological response and lowering the incidence of lung infections. Maintaining optimal vitamin D levels can be aided by getting enough sun exposure and eating foods like eggs, dairy products, fortified cereals, and fatty fish (like salmon and mackerel). However, those who are at risk of deficiency or have limited sun exposure may need to take supplements.

Zinc: Zinc has a role in the growth and operation of immune cells as well as the synthesis of antibodies, among other elements of immune function. Supplementing with zinc can assist maintain immune function, particularly in those who don't get enough zinc from their diet or who are zinc deficient. Lean meats, poultry, fish, beans, nuts, seeds, whole grains, and dairy products are among the foods high in zinc.

Probiotics: Probiotics are good microorganisms that support immune system function and gastrointestinal health. Probiotic pills may aid in maintaining a balanced gut microbiota, which is essential for immunological modulation, according to research. Eating foods high in probiotics, such tempeh, yogurt, kefir, sauerkraut, kimchi, and miso, can also supply healthy bacteria to promote immune function.

Elderberry: The fruit of the elderberry plant is used to make supplements, which are often used to enhance the immune system, especially during the cold and flu season. Antioxidant-rich and proven to have antiviral qualities, elderberries may help lessen the intensity and length of colds and influenza. To verify their effectiveness, more study is necessary.

Echinacea: Echinacea supplements are made from the plant's roots, leaves, and flowers, and they are thought to boost immunity and minimize the chance of infection. Although there have been conflicting results from certain studies indicating that echinacea may help lessen the duration of colds and flu, further research is required to confirm its efficacy.

Vitamin E: An antioxidant, vitamin E strengthens the immune system and shields cells from harm from free radicals. For those who don't receive enough vitamin E from their diet, supplements could be helpful, but it's better to obtain enough from foods like leafy greens, nuts, seeds, and vegetable oils.

Before beginning any new supplement regimen, it is imperative that you consult a healthcare provider, particularly if you are on medication, have underlying health conditions, are pregnant, or are nursing. Furthermore, supplements must to be taken in moderation and as part of a comprehensive strategy for immunological health that also includes stress management, a balanced diet, regular exercise, enough sleep, and good cleanliness.

immunological function is influenced by several elements at different phases of life, and immunological health changes over the lifespan. People can support immunological health and general well-being by taking appropriate action when they are aware of these age-related changes. An outline of immunological health during the life course is provided below:

Early Childhood and Infancy (0–2 years):

Immune system development: In the first few months of life, breast milk and maternal antibodies transmitted across the placenta provide passive immunity for infants.

Babies' immune systems grow as a result of the maturation of immune cells and the synthesis of antibodies.

Vaccinations: By promoting the development of adaptive immunity, vaccinations are essential in defending newborns and early children against infectious illnesses. Following recommended immunization regimens is vital for building immunity against numerous diseases.

Personal cleanliness and nursing: During this delicate time, exclusive breastfeeding and practicing proper cleanliness can boost an infant's immune system and lower the chance of infection.

Childhood (ages 3 to 12):

Immune system maturation: By the time a child reaches early childhood, their immune system has developed memory immune cells and produced more antibodies. Youngsters gain increased capacity to mount efficient defenses against infections.

Pathogen exposure: As children explore their surroundings, attend school, and engage with classmates, they come into contact with a variety of pathogens. The immune system is bolstered by this exposure, but infections are also more likely to occur.

Healthy lifestyle practices: Promoting healthy lifestyle practices in kids, such as eating a balanced diet, getting frequent exercise, getting enough sleep, and practicing excellent cleanliness, will strengthen their immune systems and improve their general wellbeing.

Teenage years (13–18):

Hormonal alterations: The immune system may be impacted by the hormonal changes that occur during adolescence. Hormone fluctuations may impact immunological responses and infection susceptibility.

Risk behaviors: Adolescents may partake in activities that compromise their immune systems, such as substance abuse, poor eating, and insufficient sleep. It's crucial at this point to promote healthy lifestyle choices and behaviors.

Adulthood (ages 19–64):

Immune function peak: Early to middle adulthood is often when immune function peaks. The immune systems of adults are usually well-developed and able to mount strong defenses against illnesses.

Lifestyle factors: Immune health and the prevention of chronic diseases are greatly enhanced by maintaining a healthy lifestyle, which includes eating a balanced diet, getting regular exercise, getting enough sleep, managing stress, and practicing good cleanliness.

Senior Citizens (65 and older):

Immunosenescence: Immunological system alterations brought on by aging are referred to as immunosenescence. Immune system function may deteriorate in older persons, leading to a decrease in immune cell production and a compromised ability to fight off diseases.

Immunosenescence may increase an older person's vulnerability to infections, particularly respiratory illnesses like the flu and pneumonia. It is advised that older persons receive vaccinations, such as the pneumococcal and annual flu injections, to help guard against these diseases.

Healthy aging techniques: By implementing healthy aging strategies, such as eating a balanced diet, exercising regularly, obtaining recommended vaccines, managing chronic illnesses, and keeping proper hygiene, older persons can support immunological health.

People can support immune function and advance general well-being throughout their lives by being aware of the elements that affect immunological health at various periods of life. Seeking individualised advice from healthcare specialists is also advantageous, particularly for those with underlying medical issues or unique health concerns.

CONCLUSION

To sum up, immunological health is essential to general wellbeing and vitality since it affects our capacity to fight off infections, recuperate from illnesses, and sustain ideal health for the duration of our lives. A healthy immune system is the result of a complex interaction between a number of variables, such as heredity, manner of living, environment, and medical procedures. People can strengthen immune function and foster resilience against infections and illnesses by being aware of the intricate interactions among these variables.

Immune health depends on a number of factors, including eating a nutritious, well-balanced diet, exercising frequently, getting enough sleep, controlling stress, keeping oneself clean, and abstaining from dangerous habits like smoking and binge drinking. Furthermore, maintaining current immunizations, obtaining timely medical attention when required, and placing a high priority on general wellness all support a robust and robust immune system.

It's critical to understand that a variety of environmental factors and lifestyle decisions affect immunological health rather than just one. Through a comprehensive strategy for immune support and wise health decisions, we may maximize immune performance and strengthen our capacity to flourish in the face of adversity.

In the end, making an investment in immunological health is an investment in our quality of life and long-term wellbeing. We can empower ourselves to live healthier, happier lives and lessen the toll that infectious diseases take on both individuals and communities by making immune support a priority throughout the lifetime.\

THE END